The New Comprehending

LYME DISEASE

Diet Cookbook 2024

By Sherrill Freer Smith

The material offered here is claimed to be accurate and comprehensive, and the recipient reader is totally and exclusively responsible for any liability resulting from use or misuse of any policies, processes, or instructions supplied here.

The publisher is not, under any circumstances, legally responsible or liable for any repairs, damages, or financial losses resulting directly or indirectly from the information included herein. The relevant author is the owner of all copies not owned by the publisher.

This page contains unique material that is exclusively provided for educational purposes. Information is presented for free and without any type of guarantee. The trademarks that are utilized do not get any payment, and they are published without the owner's knowledge or permission. All trade names and trademarks mentioned in the book are the sole property of their respective owners and are only used for illustration. The document does not belong to the owner.

The material offered here is claimed to be accurate and comprehensive, and the recipient reader is totally and exclusively responsible for any liability resulting from use or misuse of any policies, processes, or instructions supplied here.

The publisher is not, under any circumstances, legally responsible or liable for any repairs, damages, or financial losses resulting directly or indirectly from the information included herein. The relevant author is the owner of all copies not owned by the publisher.

This page contains unique material that is exclusively provided for educational purposes. Information is presented for free and without any type of guarantee. The trademarks that are utilized do not get any payment, and they are published without the owner's knowledge or permission. All trade names and trademarks mentioned in the book are the sole property of their respective owners and are only used for illustration. The document does not belong to the owner.

Table of Contents

What is Lyme disease?

Lyme disease is an infectious disease caused by the bacterium Borrelia burgdorferi, which is transmitted through tick bites. The infection resulting from these bites causes swelling, joint pain, rash, and flu-like symptoms. The disease can affect the nervous system, as well, causing headaches, dizziness, and other symptoms.

Lyme disease is spread by the deer tick (species Ixodes scapularis) in the northeastern United States and the western black-legged tick (species I. pacificus) in the Pacific Northwest. These ticks are typically found in wooded areas where deer are present. The tick carries the B. burgdorferi bacterium, which it passes to humans when it bites them.

Lyme disease begins with the appearance of a red spot at the site of the tick bite within days to weeks following the bite. The spot may expand into a circular or oval-shaped rash and resemble a bull's-eye: red in the center with alternating circles of white and red around it. This rash is known as erythema migrans and is unique to Lyme disease. Eventually, the rash will spread to different sites on the body. Additional symptoms include fever, aches, stiff neck, and other flu-like symptoms.

The symptoms of Lyme disease can be serious and may worsen without antibiotic treatment. Untreated cases can lead to chronic arthritis (inflammation of the joints), swelling or inflammation of the nerve that controls facial muscles, and even paralysis. Infection can spread to the spine, brain and heart as well. This can also happen if treatment is delayed or does not cure the infection.

Seek prompt medical care if you experience rash, fever, muscle aches, headache, or other symptoms of Lyme disease after being bitten by a tick.

Symptoms of Lyme disease include rash, fever, aches and swelling. You may feel like you have the flu. Left untreated, symptoms can become more serious and include joint swelling and arthritis (inflammation of the joints), especially of the knees. Lyme disease can also affect the nervous system, causing stiffness, headache, loss of muscle tone, and even paralysis.

Common symptoms of Lyme disease

Lyme disease causes symptoms that range in type and severity among individuals and may include:

- Aches
- Chills
- Decreased vision
- Fatigue
- Fever

- Headache

- Muscle pain

- Neuropathy (Bell's palsy, transverse myelitis)

- Rash, starting with a bull's-eye appearance that spreads over time

- Stiff neck

- Swelling of the knees and other large joints

- Swollen lymph nodes

Serious symptoms that might indicate a life-threatening condition

In some cases, Lyme disease can be a serious condition that should be immediately evaluated in an emergency setting. Because its symptoms can progress to serious conditions, it is important for you to be treated right away. Seek immediate medical care (call 911) for any of these serious symptoms including:

- Abnormal pupil size or nonreactivity to light

- Fever

- Heart palpitations and dizziness due to changes

  in heartbeat

- Loss of muscle tone on one or both sides of the

  face, possibly indicating paralysis

- Pain that moves from joint to joint

- Severe headaches and neck stiffness, possibly

  indicating meningitis (infection or inflammation

  of the sac around the brain and spinal cord)

- Severe swelling in the knees or joints

- Weakness or paralysis in the muscles of the

  face

One of the telltale symptoms of Lyme disease is erythema migrans, a red rash at the site of the tick bite:

- circular bull's eye tick bite rash on man's lower leg, a sign of Lyme disease

The stages of Lyme disease are progressive and depend on treatment interventions:

Early localized, just after the infection takes hold. Symptoms begin within hours, days or weeks after the tick bite, and can include skin rash—the characteristic bull's-eye rash (erythema migrans)—as well as flu-like symptoms and joint pain.

Early disseminated, occurring weeks to months after the tick bite. The bacteria are spreading further throughout the body. Because more body systems are infected, symptoms are varied and may not look related. Symptoms include eyesight problems, rash in other areas, irregular heartbeat, pain, and nerve symptoms like numbness in the arms and legs or the face.

Late disseminated stage, occurring weeks, months and extending months after the tick bite. Left untreated, Lyme disease can lead to such chronic conditions as arthritis, migraine, widespread pain, difficulty sleeping, and trouble concentrating.

Lyme disease is an infectious disease caused by the bite of a tick infected with Borrelia burgdorferi bacteria. These are in the spirochete class of bacteria, which includes the T. pallidum bacterium that causes syphilis. The deer tick in the Northeast and the western black-legged tick in the Pacific Northwest carry B. burgdorferi. The more recently discovered Borrelia mayonii can also cause Lyme disease. Transmission to humans occurs most commonly in the summer when people are most likely to be outdoors and ticks are most active.

Lyme disease bacteria usually live in rodents and other small animals and are transmitted when a tick bites an infected animal. The bacteria live in the gut of the tick. When the tick bites a human, bacteria from an infected tick can pass from the tick into the person's bloodstream.

For an infected deer tick to transmit the bacteria, it typically needs to feed for more than 36 hours. The longer the tick is attached and feeding, the greater the likelihood of the person developing Lyme disease. Rather than larger, adult ticks, smaller nymph-stage ticks (about 2 mm in diameter) cause most cases of Lyme disease because they are more likely to bite humans and are harder to detect. However, most people bitten by a tick do not develop Lyme disease.

Lyme disease symptoms typically develop between 3 and 30 days, the incubation period for B. burgdorferi. There is evidence the severity of disease and symptoms depends on the person's immune system. In other words, some people may be more at risk than others for developing Lyme disease.

It's possible to become infected a second time and develop Lyme disease again after an initial infection and treatment for Lyme disease.

A number of factors increase the risk of developing Lyme disease. Not all people with risk factors will get Lyme disease. Risk factors for Lyme disease include:

- Autoimmune disease (overactive immune response that causes the body to attack its own cells) or other conditions that compromise your immunity
- Contact with animals, especially those that are prone to tick bites
- Exposed skin unprotected by insect repellant and clothing
- Extensive time spent outdoors, especially in the spring and summer
- Extreme youth or advanced age
- Hiking or camping in tick-infested areas
- Pregnancy

Reducing your risk of Lyme disease

You may be able to lower your risk of Lyme disease by:

- Applying insect repellent containing DEET if you will be outside in areas known to have deer and black-legged ticks
- Avoiding areas of potential tick infestation
- Inspect the body for ticks when changing clothes after being outdoors (adults and children)
- Removing leaf debris, brush, and wood piles from your property
- Wearing light-colored clothing (allowing ticks to be more easily spotted and removed)
- Wearing long-sleeved shirts, tucked-in pants, and high boots if entering areas of possible infestation

To remove a tick, use fine-point tweezers to hold the tick as close to its entry point in the skin as possible. Pull back firmly in a controlled motion without jerking or twisting the tick. Gently wash the area and disinfect it with a cotton ball soaked in rubbing alcohol or an alcohol wipe.

The tick can be saved in a plastic bag for testing. However, the Centers for Disease Control and Prevention (CDC) does not recommend testing ticks for the disease. Just because a tick is carrying the disease-causing bacteria doesn't mean it has been transmitted through a bite. If the tick tests negative for bacteria, it doesn't exclude the possibility of infection from a different tick bite.

Other bacterial infections and diseases spread by ticks include:

Southern tick-associated rash illness (STARI), transmitted by the lone star tick, with symptoms including rash, fatigue, fever, headache and joint pain.

Rocky Mountain spotted fever, transmitted by the bite of a tick infected with Rickettsia bacteria, with symptoms including rash, fever and headache.

Tularemia, transmitted by ticks and deer flies infected with Francisella tularensis bacteria, with symptoms including a skin ulcer at the bite site, swollen lymph nodes, and high fever.

In addition, the nonspecific and variable nature of many Lyme disease symptoms can delay its diagnosis.

Conditions with symptoms overlapping with those of various stages of Lyme disease include chronic fatigue syndrome, fibromyalgia, mononucleosis, meningitis, septic arthritis, cancer, and lupus, among others.

An accurate diagnosis requires a physician experienced with the signs and symptoms of Lyme disease. For early Lyme disease, the most common clinical sign is the bull's eye rash (erythema migrans). The doctor also considers the patient's confirmed tick bite or probable exposure to deer ticks in a Lyme disease diagnosis. The fact that symptoms associated with Lyme disease—fatigue, difficulty concentrating, flu-like symptoms, and joint pain—overlap with several other conditions can delay diagnosis.

If the doctor is not considering the possibility of Lyme disease, it will probably not be diagnosed. If you have signs and symptoms of Lyme disease, it is fine to ask the healthcare provider, "Could this be Lyme disease?" Remember that symptoms may develop up to 30 days after the tick bite, although typically 7 to 14 days after the bite. If the problem persists and your provider is unable to determine a cause, seeking a second opinion may give you more information and answers.

A two-step blood test that detects antibodies to the bacteria is available to help confirm a Lyme disease diagnosis. Both tests must be positive to confirm Lyme disease. Results are likely to be negative the first few weeks after infection because the body has not yet built up enough antibodies for the test to detect. The Lyme disease test is most accurate a few weeks after infection.

A 10- to 14-day course of antibiotics in pill form early after infection can often cure Lyme disease. Antibiotics can also be effective in the later stages of disease, but the outcome varies among individuals. Patients in later stages of Lyme disease—those with acute joint pain or showing signs the infection has spread to the heart or central nervous system (brain and spinal cord)—may require intravenous antibiotics in a hospital.

In addition to antibiotic treatment, doctors may prescribe medicine or treatment to relieve Lyme disease symptoms, such as arthritis. You can take over-the-counter pain relievers for fever and pain.

Lyme disease recovery is usually rapid and complete, although some symptoms may recur or persist if the diagnosis is made at a later stage of the disease. It is important to follow your treatment plan for Lyme disease precisely and to take all of the antibiotics as instructed by your healthcare provider to avoid reinfection or recurrence. However, even with appropriate antibiotic treatment, the bacteria may not clear completely, and long-term and sometimes debilitating consequences are possible.

Primary care providers can treat uncomplicated cases of Lyme disease. If you have later-stage, disseminated Lyme disease, an infectious disease specialist may treat you. Other specialists you may see include a neurologist, cardiologist and rheumatologist.

Antibiotics for Lyme disease treatment

Antibiotics for Lyme disease include:

- Amoxicillin (Amoxil)

- Ceftriaxone (intravenous)

- Cefuroxime axetil (Ceftin)

- Doxycycline (Doryx)

Long-term antibiotic treatment is not more effective than the normal length of antibiotic treatment. In fact, extended antibiotic therapy can carry significant health risks, including possible bloodstream infections or heart tissue damage.

Alternative treatments for Lyme disease

Many people are interested in alternative treatments for Lyme disease. While they may help with symptoms, they do not cure the infection or the disease. Products may be labeled "natural" but that does not mean they are safe. Before you try them, confirm your diagnosis with a licensed healthcare provider with the expertise necessary to rule out other possible causes of your symptoms. Explain your interest in alternative treatment, and discuss the goals, benefits and risks of these treatments compared to traditional medicine, including antibiotics.

Alternative treatments may include:

- Acupuncture
- Herbal supplements, such as turmeric and cilantro
- Homeopathic medicine
- Medical marijuana
- Vitamin supplements
- Use caution with alternative treatments

A 2015 report identified 30 alternative therapies marketed to people who believe they have Lyme disease or some variation of it, what some people refer to as "chronic Lyme disease" or "post-Lyme disease syndrome." There are no effectiveness studies in humans for the following alternative therapies:

- Heat therapy, including lasers and Rife therapy with magnets
- Heavy metals and chelation, including removal of mercury-containing amalgam fillings and root canals
- Herbal remedies
- Oxygen therapy, including hyperbaric oxygen, ozone and hydrogen peroxide
- Pharmacological therapy

For most people with Lyme disease, treatment is successful and there is no long-term damage or complications.

Untreated Lyme disease can progress to infect multiple body systems causing significant nervous system and heart problems. The longer Lyme disease bacteria are in the body and the farther the infection spreads, the more difficult it is to cure and the greater the risk for complications and poor quality of life.

Symptoms that can last from weeks to months include:

- Severe headaches
- Severe joint pain and swelling
- Facial palsy
- Lyme carditis (heart infection)

- Decreased vision (macular edema, uveitis, retinal inflammation)
- Shortness of breath
- Meningitis or encephalitis
- Neuropathy
- Thinking and memory problems

After antibiotic treatment for Lyme disease, up to 10% of patients develop post-treatment Lyme disease syndrome (PTLDS or PLDS). PTLDS can persist for many months. Signs and symptoms of PTLDS are similar to early-stage Lyme disease and include fatigue and joint and muscle aches and pains. Patients also report difficulty sleeping, memory problems, and headache.

Some people use the term chronic Lyme disease to describe a condition marked by symptoms like Lyme disease, such as fatigue, pain, memory problems, and arthritis. However, in many of these cases, lab tests for current or past Lyme disease are negative. For this reason, Lyme disease experts support no longer using the term chronic Lyme disease.

What are the potential complications of Lyme disease?

Most cases of Lyme disease can be cured with antibiotics, especially if treatment is begun early in the course of illness. However, a small percentage of people with Lyme disease have symptoms that last for months to years after treatment with antibiotics.

Complications of Lyme disease range from joint pain and stiffness to meningitis (infection or inflammation of the sac around the brain and spinal cord) and paralysis. About 10 to 20% of untreated or complicated cases of Lyme disease can progress to arthritis.

You can help minimize your risk of serious complications by following the treatment plan you and your healthcare professional design specifically for you. Complications of Lyme disease include:

- Arthritis
- Cognitive deficits (for example, memory loss and shorter attention span)
- Fatigue
- Meningitis (infection or inflammation of the sac around the brain and spinal cord)
- Muscle and joint pain
- Paralysis
- Permanent vision loss
- Sleep disturbances

In rare cases, Lyme disease can be fatal. The most serious threat comes from Lyme disease bacteria entering heart tissue. This is Lyme carditis, which affects about 1% of people with Lyme disease. The infection can disrupt the heart's electrical system causing heart block, which can be fatal if not recognized and treated rapidly.

Lyme disease awareness

The number of Lyme disease cases has been increasing over the last 25 years. Improvements in prevention will help control these numbers. To prevent Lyme disease, avoid areas known to harbor infected ticks, use insect repellent, perform a body check after being outdoors, and remove ticks as soon as possible. A Lyme disease vaccine was approved in

1998; however, sales decreased significantly and the company stopped making it in 2002. Research is underway on newer types of Lyme disease vaccines.

May is Lyme disease awareness month. Learn more about Lyme disease awareness at Global Lyme Alliance and Lyme disease research efforts at the CDC.

Lyme disease is a bacterial infection caused by the bacterium Borrelia burgdorferi. It is spread through the bite of infected ticks.

Ticks are very small, and their bites—which can occur anywhere on the body—are usually painless, so you may not immediately be aware that you have been bitten. In most cases, the tick must be attached to the body for 24 hours before Lyme disease is transmitted.

The signs and symptoms of Lyme disease usually start within three to 30 days after you've been bitten by an infected tick. Many people experience flu-like symptoms after being bitten, while more serious symptoms show up weeks after the bite. Early signs and symptoms of Lyme disease include:

- Chills

- Fatigue

- Fever

- Headache

- Joint and muscle aches

- Rash (shaped like a bullseye)

- Swollen lymph nodes

If left untreated, symptoms can worsen to include Bell's palsy (facial paralysis), severe headaches, muscle, joint, and tendon pain, cardiac (heart) problems, and neurological disorders.

Most cases of Lyme disease can be managed and treated with two to three weeks of antibiotics. Depending on the severity of your symptoms and how long after the bite you were diagnosed, you may need a longer course of antibiotics to clear up the infection.

Many people turn to natural remedies to help treat Lyme disease.

Essential Oils for Lyme Disease

It is believed that many essential oils have antimicrobial activities, and some people with persistent Lyme disease symptoms have turned to essential oils to help reduce symptoms of the disease.

Researchers tested 34 essential oils against B. burgdorferi in the lab (not in humans) and found cinnamon bark, clove bud, citronella, wintergreen, and oregano show strong activity against the bacterium that causes Lyme disease, even more effectively than daptomycin, the "gold standard" antibiotic many people with Lyme disease are prescribed.

These results indicate that essential oils show promise as treatments for persistent Lyme disease, but clinical trials are needed in order to show their effectiveness in humans.

When used properly, most essential oils are safe and free of adverse side effects. However, it is important to use them carefully. They can irritate the skin if not properly diluted, and some should not be taken internally.

Purchase high-quality essential oils that go through testing to ensure the product is safe to use. Follow the usage and dilution instructions on the label carefully. Talk with your healthcare professional before using essential oils to avoid drug interactions with any medications you are taking.

Naturopathic Treatment

Naturopathic treatment for Lyme disease takes a whole-body approach. Your naturopathic practitioner will evaluate your diet, lifestyle, immune status, environment, and any other medical conditions you have to come up with a treatment plan.

Licensed naturopathic practitioners who are able to prescribe pharmaceuticals may use antibiotic treatment in combination with natural approaches.

Your naturopathic Lyme disease treatment may include a combination of nutritional and lifestyle counseling, homeopathic remedies, herbs, and dietary supplements that are recommended based on your specific symptoms and needs.

The goal is to support your body's immune system, promote healthy detoxification, and protect and repair the body. Many people choose to seek naturopathic treatment as a complementary therapy and follow the recommended protocol in combination with antibiotic medication that has been prescribed by their primary care physician or other healthcare provider.

Research on the efficacy of naturopathic treatment for Lyme disease is limited.

Herbs for Lyme Disease Treatment

Herbs have been used as a medicinal treatment for thousands of years. Many people have turned to herbal remedies to help provide relief from Lyme disease when antibiotics didn't completely help eliminate symptoms.

One research study found that a combination of doxycycline (antibiotic) and baicalein (the active ingredient found in Chinese skullcap) provides additional healing benefits.5 According to a 2020 laboratory study, seven herbal medicines have been shown to kill B. burgdorferi in test tubes:

- Cryptolepis sanguinolenta
- Juglans nigra (black walnut)
- Polygonum cuspidatum (Japanese knotweed)
- Artemisia annua (sweet wormwood)
- Uncaria tomentosa (cat's claw)
- Cistus incanus
- Scutellaria baicalensis (Chinese skullcap)

Garlic has antibacterial effects and may help prevent tick bites. One study determined that people who took garlic supplements reported fewer tick bites than the placebo group. Garlic essential oil has been shown to eliminate the bacterium that causes Lyme disease.

Garlic can interact with certain medications, so speak with your healthcare provider before using it to prevent or treat Lyme disease.

Stevia—a natural sweetener and sugar substitute derived from the leaves of the Stevia rebaudiana plant—may be effective in treating Lyme disease. A study published in the European Journal of Microbiology and Immunology discovered that stevia extracts are more effective in killing Lyme disease bacterium in the lab (not tested in humans) than the standard antibiotics.

Chelation Therapy

Chelation therapy is a method that involves removing heavy metals from the bloodstream. Some people believe that Lyme disease symptoms are linked to heavy metal toxicity in the body caused by environmental factors (e.g., pollution, lead exposure) and turn to chelation therapy to treat Lyme disease.

A chelating agent is a molecule that binds with heavy metals in the body and eliminates them through the kidneys. Chelation therapy may be given as an oral preparation or by intravenously administering saline and a chelating agent such as ethylenediaminetetraacetic acid (EDTA).

Chelation therapy is approved by the Food and Drug Administration when administered by a licensed practitioner. It is used to treat lead poisoning. Some alternative practitioners use it for additional applications, including atherosclerosis and arthritis.

There is currently no evidence to suggest that Lyme disease is caused by or worsened by heavy metal exposure, and chelation therapy is not a proven treatment for Lyme disease.

Other Natural Treatments

There are many natural treatment options offered to treat Lyme disease. A 2015 study identified 30 alternative treatments, including:

- Acupuncture
- Bee venom
- Energy and radiation-based therapies
- Enemas
- Magnets

- Nutritional therapy

- Photon therapy

- Sauna

- Stem cell transplantation

There is currently no research to prove the efficacy of these unconventional treatments, and in some cases, the treatments may be more harmful than helpful.

Lyme Bay brill with crusted almond, lobster and linguin

Ingredients

- 4 x 170 g brill portions

- 100 g roasted and crushed almonds

- 12 bok choi leaves

- 1 lobster, cooked and cleaned

- 4 portions of linguine (or your favourite pasta)

- 1 shallot, chopped

- 5 button mushrooms, sliced

- 200 ml lobster stock

- 50 ml sweet wine

- 25 ml brand

- 100 ml whipping cream

- 30 g butter

- a small handful of fermented wild garlic

Method

- Sweat the shallot and mushroom until soft.

- Add the sweet wine and brandy and reduce by half.

- Add the lobster stock and further reduce by one third, then add the cream, bring to the boil and season.

- Sear the bill fillets in a non-stick pan for two to three minutes on each side.

- Cover with the crushed almonds and bake carefully under a grill until golden brown.

- Grill the lobster meat until warmed through.

- Place the cooked pasta in the centre of the bowl and cover generously with the lobster sauc

- Add the fermented wild garlic, bok choi leaves, grilled lobster and brill.

1. **Coconut Cranberry Almond Butter Rice Cakes**

Ingredients

- brown rice cakes
- Tbsp. well-stirred creamy almond butter
- 1/4 tsp. coconut flakes
- 2 Tbsp. dried cranberries
- 1 Tbsp. finely chopped fresh basil
- 2 tsp. pumpkin seeds
- 1/4 tsp. fresh lemon zest

Instructions

- Lay rice cakes on a flat surface. Spread almond butter onto each rice cake using a knife. Top with remaining ingredients.
- Serve immediately.

Nutrition Tips Facts

Coconut Cranberry Almond Butter Rice Cakes

- Calories 250Calories from Fat 144
- % Daily Value*
- Fat 16g25%
- Saturated Fat 2g13%
- Sodium 5mg0%
- Potassium 254mg7%
- Carbohydrates 25g8%
- Fiber 4g17%
- Sugar 11g12%
- Protein 7g14%
- Vitamin A 390IU8%
- Vitamin C 2mg2%
- Calcium 90mg9%
- Iron 2mg11%
- Percent Daily Values are based on a 2000 calorie diet.

Tick Bite Prevention Body Oil

Ingredients

- 4 oz carrier oil of choice
- 8 drops each of these tick-repelling essential oils (vetiver, clove, oregano, and spearmint)

Instructions

Blend, pour into a glass spritzer bottle, and spray periodically to ankles, arms, etc

Super Healthy Green Smoothie

Ingredients

- cups romaine lettuce (or other green such as spinach or arugula)
  - stalks celery
- 1/2 cucumber
- 1 avocado

- 1.5 carrots

- 1 orange

- 1/4 cup parsley

- 6-10 ounces water

Instructions

Place all ingredients in blender and blend at high power. Enjoy!

DIY Tick Repellent Spra

Ingredients

- tablespoons dried lavender

- tablespoons dry sage

- tablespoons dry thyme

- tablespoons dry rosemary

- 15 drops of peppermint essential oil or 1 tablespoon dried mint

- 32 ounces of quality apple cider vinegar

Salmon Ginger Tamari Stir-Fry

Ingredients

- 1 lb. wild salmon, skinless and cut into cubes
- 1 tbs sesame oil
- 1 organic red pepper, sliced
- 1 organic yellow pepper, sliced
- 1 head of organic broccoli, including stem, cut into florets, stem peeled and sliced
- heads or organic baby bok choy, rough chopped
- oz. shiitake mushrooms, sliced
- 1 package of brown rice noodles

Instructions

- Start making the sauce by combining all of the ingredients except for the brown rice flour into a bowl.

- Place the salmon into a separate bowl, add in enough sauce to just cover the salmon. Cover and place in fridge while you prep the veggies.Cook salmon in a teaspoon of sesame oil on medium heat. Flip once. Should only take a few minutes. Once it starts to flake, remove from pan.Boil water for the noodles, cook according to instructions on the package.

- Add the remaining sauce to a sauce pan. Whisk in one tablespoon of brown rice flour and bring to a boil. Once it starts to thicken, remove from heat Add in all veggies except for the bok choy into the pan the salmon was in with whatever liquid was left over. Cover for a few minutes.Once the veggies are slightly tender, add in the bok choy, a few tablespoons of sauce, and the cooked noodles. Stir gently so everything is coated. Place salmon on top, and dinner is ready.

Natural Tick Repellent

Ingredients

- ⅓ cup of distilled water
- ¼ cup of witch hazel
- 30 drops of your preferred essential oil (tick-repelling essential oils: lemongrass, peppermint, geranium, and cedarwood)

Instructions

- Take a glass jar (label it so that it's not used for food or drinks) and add ⅓ cup of distilled water. Next, add ¼ cup of witch hazel.

- Add 30 drops of your preferred essential oil (if you're using two, add 15 drops of each essential oil, and ten drops of each oil if you're using three).
- Screw on the lid tightly and shake the jar vigorously. Transfer the contents of the jar to a spray bottle, and you're good to go!
- Repellent spray tip: The key to adequate protection is to reapply frequently. As soon as the scent wears off from the spray so has the effectiveness, so it's important to keep reapplying. Every one to two hours is recommended.
- Note: You can tweak this recipe to fit your own bug-repelling needs.

Bay lobster salad with crispy bacon

Ingredients

- 1 lobster, cooked (Mark uses Lyme Bay lobsters)
- bacon rashers, sliced into lardons
- handfuls of salad leaves, Mark uses a mix of Vietnamese coriander, nasturtium leaves, New Zealand spinach, oxeye daisy leaves and celery leaves
- 1/2 tsp Tewkesbury mustard
- 2 tbsp of cold-pressed rapeseed oil, Mark uses Hillfarm
- 1 tbsp of vinegar, ideally homemade (see recipe) or from a good quality bottle of cider vinegar
- freshly ground black pepper

Carrot Almond Pancakes

Ingredients

- 1 cup peeled and grated carrots (2-3 carrots)
- ¼ cup almonds
- 1 slice fresh ginger (1/8-inch thick)
- 1 teaspoon ground flaxseed
- tablespoons unsweetened shredded coconut
- ½ teaspoon ground cinnamon
- 1 egg
- ¼ teaspoon sea salt
- ½ teaspoon vanilla
- 1-2 tablespoons Ghee (page 234)
- 1 teaspoon raw honey
- Blueberriess

Instructions

Place the grated carrots in a medium-sized bowl.

Place the almonds, ginger and flaxseed in the bowl of a food processor. Pulse 5-6 times until the almonds are finely ground.

Add the almond mixture and all of the remaining ingredients, except for the ghee, honey and blueberries, to the grated carrots.

Heat the ghee in a small frying pan over medium heat for 2 minutes, or until hot.

Pour two ¼-cup portions of pancake batter into the frying pan, and cook for about 3 minutes per side, or until lightly browned. Repeat with the remaining batter.

Top with honey and blueberries if desired, and serve hot

Gluten Free Pasta Puttanesca

Ingredients

12 oz Gluten Free Pasta 1 tablespoon olive oil

cloves of garlic

1/3 cup chopped flat leaf parsley

1/3 cup kalamata olives

tablespoons of capers

1 1/2 tsp anchovy paste

1 1/2 tsp dried oregano

1/4 tsp of crushed red pepper

1 (28oz) can diced tomatoes

Directions

Bring a large pot of water to a boil

Add pasta and cook to your liking

While that's cooking, heat oil over medium heat

Add garlic and saute for a minute

Add parsley, olives, capers, paste, oregano, crushed red pepper and saute for another 1 -2 minutes

Add tomatoes and simmer for a few more minutes

Drain your pasta, add it to your sauce.

Ham Nectarine & Spring Mix Pizza

Ingredients

1 flatout wrap

1/4 cup cooked ham

1/2 diced nectarine

1-2 handful spring mix/spinach

T mozzarella cheese shredded

Instructions

Preheat oven to 350 degrees

Slice and dice your nectarine and ham if not already done

Have however many flatout wraps as you desire and then build your pizza with the above ingredients however you would like!

Place on a cookie sheet and bake for ~11 minutes or until crispy and the cheese is melted

Eat and enjoy!

White Gate Farm's Fennel Vichyssoise

Ingredients

large bulbs fennel cores removed and sliced thickly

cups peeled and finely diced raw potatoes

2 medium onions peeled and chopped roughly

cloves garlic peeled and sliced in half

tablespoons butter

3 cups organic chicken stock

1 teaspoon salt

1 teaspoon freshly ground white pepper

1-1/2 cups (or more) organic heavy cream

Finely sliced scallions, chopped chives and/or cucumber for garnish

Instructions

Toss fennel with olive oil to coat and a little salt. Roast in a 400 degree oven for about 30 minutes until lightly brown.

Cook the potatoes in salted water to cover until just tender.

Melt the butter in a skillet and cool the onions and garlic gently, tossing them lightly, for a few minutes. Add the chicken broth and bring to a boil. Lower the heat, add roasted fennel and simmer with the onions and garlic until tender. Strain the potatoes, add to the broth mixture and season to taste with salt, pepper. Put this in the blender (you will need to blend it in two lots) and blend for 1 minute, or until smooth. Chill.

When ready to serve, mix in heavy cream in half cup measurements until desired consistency. Taste and re-season with salt and white pepper if necessary.

Garnish with scallions, chives and cucumber.

Heather's christmas cake recipe

Ingredients

10oz currants

12oz sultanas

3oz dried cherries

1 lemon (zest and juice)

1 orange (zest and juice)

2tbsp spiced rum

1tsp mixed spice

1/2 tsp cinnamon

1tbsp cherry jam

5oz butter

6oz soft brown sugar

4 eggs

7oz plain flour

Directions

In a large saucepan add the currants, sultanas, dried cherries, orange zest and juice, lemon zest and juice, rum, mixed spice, cinnamon, jam, butter and sugar. Cook together on a medium heat for 10 minutes, stirring regularly so that it doesn't burn on the bottom and all the sugar and butter melt and coat the fruit.

Take off the heat and leave to cool for 30 minutes.

Whilst the ingredients are cooling, spend some time lining your 8" round tin. As laborious and fiddly as this step is, it is well worth the effort as it helps stop the edges from drying out. Line the insides with 2 layers of baking parchment. Then take some brown paper and line the outside of the tin, making sure to have a couple of inches above the tin too, and tie with string to secure.

Preheat the oven to 140 fan/gas mark 1.

Once the fruit mixture has cooled, carefully stir in the eggs. Then stir in the flour.

Place the mixture in the tin and then bake in the oven for 2.5 hours. Check the cake every 15-30 minutes after the initial 2.5 hours, until a skewer inserted into the middle of the cake comes out clean. Allow the cake to cool in the tin.

Once cold, the cake can be covered with a layer of marzipan and icing ready for Christmas Day. If you have made the cake in advance, once the cake is cold, wrap the cake in a layer of baking parchment, a layer of foil and place in an airtight container. You can bake up to 3 months in advance and keep the cake in this way. About 1 week before Christmas, you can ice the cake however you fancy. If you would like to – every 2 weeks, poke the cake a number of times with a skewer and spoon over some more rum. This is called 'feeding' the cake (and it also makes the cake slightly alcoholic so be careful if you know children will be eating the cake!

Knotweed Gin And Tonic

Ingredients

ounces knotweed infused gin (see note)

4-5 ounces tonic water

a few ice cubes, ideally made with tonic water

Instructions

Mix the ingredients in the glass and give it a stir.

Garnish with fresh knotweed stalk (optional).

Enjoy!.

Life-Changing Green Drink

Ingredients

1 (packed) c. dark greens (any you like, including kale, chard, spinach, mustard greens, dandelion greens, etc.)

1 handful parsley

1 handful cilantro

8 fresh basil leaves (optional)

1 small apple

1/2 lemon or lime

1-2 c . water , as needed for blending

Instructions

Blend all until smooth (1-2 minutes).

Notes

Fat: 0.7 g Carbs: 28.5 g Sugar: 19.5 g Protein: 2.3 g; Nutrition facts based on using one cup spinach, 1/3 cup parsley, 1/3 cup cilantro, and one lemon wedge. WW points (new system):

Nutrition

Calories: 113kcal

Spiced Chickpea & Carrot Salad with Ancient Grains

Ingredients

2/3 cup cooked millet

¾ cup cooked chickpeas

¾ cup mixed shredded cabbage

1 carrot cut into ribbons

1/3 cup chopped red pepper

tbsp olive oil

1 tsp lime juice

1 tsp cinnamon

1 tsp cumin

1 tsp mint

Instructions

Combine the olive oil, lime juice and spices in a
large bowl and mix well

Add remaining ingredients and stir to evenly
coat

Let stand for at least 30 minutes before serving

Recipe Notes

If your using canned chickpeas rinse them well under cool water first. For the cabbage mix I find it easiest to use the pre-chopped bags of mixed cabbage or even broccoli slaw will work. The carrot can be easily sliced into ribbons using a regular vegetable peeler – just peel the outer edges, discard them and continue to peel the carrot lengthwise into long ribbons.

Fillet of Lyme Bay red gurnard escabeche

Ingredients

Red gurnard

fillets of red gurnard (pin-boned)

1 head garlic, peeled and sliced

sprigs lemon thyme

150ml extra virgin olive oil

50ml fresh lemon juice

Escabeche

200g carrots peeled and finely sliced

2 small onions peeled and finely sliced

1 clove chopped garlic

50ml white wine vinegar

75g white wine

100g olive oil

2g coriander seeds crushed

A pinch of saffron - powder works best

Method

In a shallow container, combine the olive oil, garlic, lemon juice and lemon thyme. Then, season the red gurnard with a little Cornish sea salt and ground white pepper, while you bring a frying pan up to a high heat. Pan-fry the fillets in a little of the olive oil, approximately 3 minutes on the skin side, 1 minute on the flesh. Once cooked, remove and place into the container of the remaining ingredients and leave to infuse.

For the escabeche, gently sweat the onion and garlic in the olive oil in a low heat so it cooks without colour. Add the carrot and once both are just cooked, add all the remaining ingredients. Allow the mixture to come to the boil, then remove from the heat.

To serve, spoon the escabeche in the centre of the plate, then place the red gurnard on top. Finish with a little dressed salad. Enjoy.

Conclusion

There is no particular cause or indication of nervous system infection associated with Lyme disease.72 Individuals who do not have Lyme disease may experience the same incapacitating symptoms, such as extreme exhaustion and problems with cognition. This condition was formerly known as chronic fatigue syndrome, but it has lately been proposed to rename it "systemic exertion intolerance disease."1. The latter is genuine, debilitating, and seems to accompany a variety of diseases, including perhaps Lyme disease. However, there is no proof that it is brought on by persistent infection with B. burgdorferi, other tick-borne pathogens, or any other pathogen that has not yet been identified. Antibiotic therapy of this symptom complex has a significant risk but is unlikely to benefit patients.